Dash Diet

Recipes and Beginner's Guide

The Best Dash Diet Recipes to lower Blood Pressure and to keep you Fit and Healthy!

Contents

Introduction

I want to thank and congratulate you for downloading the book "*25 Dash Diet Recipes and Beginner's Guide: The Best Dash Diet Recipes to lower Blood Pressure and to keep you Fit and Healthy!*"

If you're curious about what the DASH Diet is about and how you can incorporate it in your life, now's your chance to do so!

With the help of this book, you will not only get to learn more about the Dash Diet, you'll also learn 25 exciting DASH Diet recipes that you can make for breakfast, lunch, dinner, snacks and desserts, as well. Plus, you'll be able to learn the best tips about how you can make the diet really work for you and which foods you're supposed to eat or use for cooking. By the end of this book, you'll no longer be clueless about the DASH diet and you'll be able to boost your cooking skills, too!

What are you waiting for? Start reading this book now and be the healthiest version of you that you can be!

Once again, thank you and enjoy!

Chapter 1: DASH Diet Beginner's Guide

A lot of people are getting curious about the DASH Diet and have wanted to try it. So, what exactly is the DASH Diet?

The DASH Diet was developed with the help of the US National Institute of Health as a means to lower blood pressure without the need for medication. DASH actually stands for Dietary Approaches to Stop Hypertension. Aside from being able to lower blood pressure, DASH Diet has also proven to lower the risk of other diseases such as stroke, heart failure, diabetes, cancer, osteoporosis, and kidney stones. Not only will it work for you today, it's designed in such a way that it will have long term effects—so you can be sure that you'll be able to live a long and healthy life.

The Dash Diet is comprised of low-fat or non-fat dairy, fruits, vegetables, lean meats, whole grains, poultry, fish, beans, and nuts that are filled with various vitamins and minerals such as potassium, magnesium and calcium that your body certainly needs to grow. It is a diet that is high in fiber and low in fat so it would be easy for you to lose weight and lower your cholesterol levels and it also aims to reduce the amount of sodium that you consume so the systems of the body can be stabilized. This way, you can live your life the best way possible. Aside from eating the right kinds of food, it is also recommended that you lessen or quit smoking and exercise regularly so you could be sure that you'd be able to maintain your ideal weight and that a lot of diseases could be prevented.

If you choose to follow the DASH diet, your systolic blood pressure will be able to drop by at least 7 to 12 points, which is a big help for your cholesterol levels to go down and make sure that you would not be suffering from any heart ailments or strokes anytime soon.

To help you understand the diet better, here's a simple chart about how much of these various food products you should take on a 2000 calorie diet.

Food Types	Number of Servings (per week) on a 2000 Calorie Diet
Fruits	4 to 5
Grains/Grain Products	7 to 8
Legumes, Seeds and Nuts	4 to 5
Low-Fat/Non-Fat Dairy	2 to 3
Poultry, Fish and Lean Meats	1 to 2
Sweets/Fats	1 to 2
Vegetables	4 to 5

A few reminders:

1. Grains can be eaten for most of the day because they are rich in fiber and low in fat. Make sure to look for those that are labeled "100 percent whole wheat" or "100 percent whole grain".
2. You can use both fresh and frozen vegetables—not just as side dishes, but as main meals. You'll find some recipes in the next chapters that makes use of vegetables.
3. It's also good to eat edible fruit or vegetable peels, because they have a lot of fiber. Good examples include peels of apples and pears and other fruits with pits.
4. Check nutritional labels to make sure that you choose products that have no sugar in them, if choosing canned fruits.
5. If you're suffering from some diseases, check with your doctor first if it's safe to eat citrus fruits as they may counteract some medications.
6. If you're lactose-intolerant, make sure that you choose only lactose-free products.
7. Don't eat regular kinds of cheese too much as they are loaded with sodium.
8. Fat-free or low-fat yogurt will help you curb those dairy cravings. Yogurt's healthy and can be considered as a sweet treat, too. It's best added with fruits, which you'll also be learning about later.
9. If you really love sweets, make sure to choose those that are low-fat or fat-free such as jelly beans, fruit ices, sorbets, or graham crackers. Make sure to check nutritional labels for added sugar. Avoid products with added sugar as much as possible.
10. Always make sure that you skin meat, poultry and fish and that you bake instead of frying.
11. Tempeh or Tofu are good meat alternatives because they are soy-based and don't contain much fat.
12. Tuna, herring, and salmon are the best kinds of fish out there, when fiber content is concerned.
13. Make sure not to drink too much alcohol as this increases blood pressure. You can drink coffee but make sure to keep it under control.
14. As much as possible, don't use too much salt in your recipes and make sure to buy foods that are labeled as "very low sodium", "sodium free", or "no salt added".
15. And, don't forget to exercise! Joining DASH Diet support groups might be helpful, too.

Now that you know what and how much you should eat, it's time to get in the kitchen and start cooking!

Chapter 1: DASH Diet Recipes for Breakfast

1. Amazing Breakfast Pudding

Ingredients:

-4 eggs
-3 cups whole wheat bread, cubed
-1 ½ cups low fat milk
-1/2 tsp ground cinnamon
-1/2 tsp vanilla extract
-1/2 cup apple, peeled and diced
-1/8 tsp salt
-2 tsp powdered sugar
-1/2 cup raisins

Procedure:
Preheat the oven to 350 °F.

Then, combine eggs, vanilla, brown sugar, salt, and cinnamon in a large bowl and whisk all the ingredients together thoroughly.

Next, add diced apple, bread cubes, and raisins. Mix all the ingredients together until well-combined or until the bread has been soaked in the liquid before coating a baking dish with baking spray. Then, move the bread mixture into a pan and cover it with foil. Refrigerate overnight.

Bake the pudding for around 40 minutes then check if it has turned golden brown. After doing so, put it back in the oven and bake for another 20 minutes.

Allow the mixture to cool for around 10 minutes and then serve dusted with powdered sugar. Enjoy!

Total Calories: 250

2. Cheesy Mini Egg Omelets with Broccoli

Ingredients:

-1 cup egg whites
-4 cups broccoli florets
-1/2 cup Parmesan Cheese, grated
-1/2 cup reduced fat Cheddar
-cooking spray
-salt
-fresh pepper
-1 Tbsp Olive Oil

Procedure:

Preheat the oven to 350 °F while steaming the broccoli. Steam it for around 6 to 7 minutes. Once it's done, mash the broccoli into smaller pieces then mix it with salt, pepper, and olive oil.

Then, spray a muffin tin with some cooking spray and add the broccoli mixture.

Beat eggs, egg whites, salt, pepper, and Parmesan Cheese in a bowl and pour this mixture into the muffin tin. Add grated cheese on top and bake for around 20 minutes or until cooked.

Once done, serve immediately and enjoy!

Total Calories: 104

3. Scrambled Mushroom, Spinach, and Feta Cheese

Ingredients:

-1 cup chopped fresh spinach
-1/2 cup sliced fresh mushrooms
-2 Tbsp feta cheese
-1 whole egg
-2 egg whites
-pepper, to taste
-cooking spray

Procedure:

Spray a pan with cooking spray and heat it over medium heat. Add spinach and mushrooms and sauté until spinach is wilted or for around 2 to 3 minutes.

Next, whisk egg whites and 1 whole egg in a bowl together with pepper and feta cheese. Pour this mixture over the vegetables and cook until eggs are cooked through or for around 3 to 4 minutes.

Serve immediately.

Total Calories: 150

4. The Very Best Granola

Ingredients:

-4 Tbsp honey
-1/4 cup canola oil
-1 cup almonds, slivered
-6 cups rolled oats
1 ½ tsp vanilla
-1 cup raisins
-3/4 cup walnuts, chopped
-2 cups bran flakes
-1/2 cup shredded unsweetened coconut
-cooking spray

Procedure:

Preheat the oven to 325 °F.

Then, mix honey, oil, and vanilla altogether in a pan. Stir for around 5 minutes and cook over low heat. Mix thoroughly.

Put all of the ingredients with the exception of the raisins in a large bowl. Mix until well-combined then add the honey and oil mixture that you have made earlier. Make sure that the grains get to be well-coated.

Use some cooking spray to spray a baking tray with and cover it with parchment paper. Place the cereal in the said tray and bake for around 25 minutes or until lightly browned. Make sure to stir whenever possible so burning could be prevented.

Take out the cereal from the oven and let it cool. Serve topped with raisins and enjoy!

Total Calories: 200

5. Nutty Banana Pancakes

Ingredients:

-1/4 tsp cinnamon
-1 cup whole wheat flour
-1 cup 1% or low fat milk
-1 large banana, mashed
-1/4 tsp salt
-2 Tbsp walnuts, chopped
-1 tsp vanilla
-2 tsp oil
-3 large egg whites
-2 tsp baking powder

Procedure:

Combine oil, egg white, milk, mashed bananas, and vanilla in another bowl and mix until smooth.

Next, combine all of the wet ingredients together and mix them with the dry ingredients. Use a spoon to mix them until you can no longer see and feel any dry spots.

Pour at least ¼ cup of the batter onto a griddle and then flip the pancakes once bubbles have formed. Repeat process with the rest of the batter.

Serve and enjoy!

Total Calories: 146

Chapter 2: DASH Diet Recipes for Lunch

6. Grilled Vegetable Sandwich

Ingredients:

-1 Tbsp lemon juice
-3 cloves garlic, minced
-3 Tbsp light mayonnaise
-2 slices focaccia bread
-1 small yellow squash, sliced
-1 red onion, sliced
-1 small zucchini, sliced
-1 cup reduced fat feta cheese, crumbled
-1 cup red bell peppers, sliced
-1/8 cup olive oil

Procedure:

Mix garlic, mayonnaise, and lemon juice in a bowl and then keep it in the fridge and then preheat the grill in high heat.

Next, brush each side of the vegetables with oil and arrange the vegetables on the grill. Place zucchini in the middle, next to the bell peppers and arrange squash and onions around them. Cook each side for three minutes or until peppers have been cooked.

Spread cut sides of the bread with mayonnaise and put feta cheese on top. Put these on the grill, cheese side up, and cover for at least 2 to 3 minutes.

After grilling, layer bread around the vegetables and serve.

Total Calories: 240

7. Jolly Veggie Wraps

Ingredients:

-4 large lettuce leaves, washed and then patted dry
-1/2 cup celery, diced
-1 large chicken breast
-1/4 cup onion, minced
-2/3 cup mandarin oranges, drained
-1 tsp soy sauce
-2 Tbsp mayonnaise
-1/4 tsp black pepper
-1/4 tsp garlic powder
-1 large whole wheat tortilla

Procedure:

Cook chicken breast in a non-stick pan over high heat until heated through. After cooking, cut chicken into ½ inch cubes.

Mix celery, chicken, onions, and oranges in a medium bowl then add garlic, soy sauce, pepper and mayonnaise. Mix these ingredients together until chicken is well-coated.

Next, place the tortilla on a large plate or on a cutting board, cut it into quarters, and place a lettuce leaf on each tortilla. Make sure to trim the leaves so they won't look messy over the tortilla.

In the middle of each leaf, put ¼ of the chicken mixture then roll each tortilla into the shape of a cone.

Serve like sandwich wraps and enjoy!

Total Calories: 192

8. Healthy Tuna Melt

Ingredients:

-1/4 cup onion, chopped
-1/3 cup celery, chopped
-6 oz tuna, packed in water, drained
-3 oz grated reduced fat cheddar
-2 split whole wheat English Muffins
-1/4 cup Thousand Island or Russian dressing
-1/4 cup onion, chopped
-black pepper and salt, to taste

Procedure:

Preheat the broiler and mix celery and tuna with the salad dressing.

Season the mixture with salt and black pepper while toasting the English Muffins.

Put the muffins on a baking tray, split side up together with ¼ of the tuna mixture. Broil until heated through or for around 2 to 3 minutes and then add cheese on top.

Broil again for a minute or until cheese melts.

Serve and enjoy!

Total Calories: 210

9. Pita Pizza Surprise

Ingredients:

-1/2 cup sodium mozzarella cheese, grated
-2 pieces whole wheat pita bread
-vegetables, such as onions, bell peppers, mushrooms, artichoke hearts, olives, etc.
-1/4 cup pizza sauce

Procedure:

Preheat the oven to 350 °F then cut the pita bread in half. Add cheese, pizza sauce, and vegetables inside.

After stuffing the pita, wrap it with aluminum foil and bake until cheese melts or for around 7 to 10 minutes.

Now, you have some healthy pizza with you. Enjoy!

Total Calories: 170

10. Amazing Vegetable Quesadillas served with Yogurt and Cilantro Dip

Ingredients:

-2 Tbsp cilantro, chopped
-6 soft corn tortillas
-1 cup black beans
-1/2 cup corn kernels
-1/2 bell pepper, chopped finely
-1 medium carrot, shredded
-1/2 Jalapeno Pepper, minced finely
-1 cup low-fat cheese, shredded
For the dip:
-2 Tbsp cilantro, chopped finely
-1 cup plain non-fat yogurt
-juice from ½ lime

Procedure:

In low heat, preheat a large skillet.

Arrange 3 tortillas and divide corn, cheese, beans, peppers and carrots over the tortillas. Place another tortilla on top of the first tortilla then put the tortilla in a skillet.

Warm tortilla until cheese melts or for around 3 minutes. This will also make the tortilla golden.

Cook each side for a minute then mix lime juice, cilantro, and yogurt in a bowl.

Next, cut each of the quesadillas into 4 wedges so you'd have a total of 12 wedges. Serve 3 wedges on each plate with the yogurt-cilantro dip.

Enjoy!

Reminder: If there are any leftovers, make sure to refrigerate them within 2 hours.

Total Calories: 240

Chapter 3: DASH Diet Recipes for Dinner

11.   Sausage and Brazilian Black Beans

Ingredients:

-8 oz low fat Polish sausage, cut into small pieces
-1 can black beans, drained and rinsed
-2 cups water
-2 tsp vegetable oil
-1 clove garlic, minced
-1 large onion, chopped
-1 cup uncooked brown rice
-1 tsp ground cumin
-1 red bell pepper, chopped

Procedure:

Over medium heat, heat some oil and then sauté onions and sausages until onions are transparent.

Next, add the rest of the ingredients and broil the mixture over high heat. After doing so, reduce heat to low and simmer for around 40 minutes.

You may also add mushrooms to make it tastier. Adding Cayenne Pepper is also encouraged.

Serve and enjoy!

Total Calories: 190

12.　　　Avocado and Orange Chicken

Ingredients:

-4 skinless and boneless chicken breasts
1/4 cup red onion, minced
-1 cup low fat yogurt
-salt
-1 Tbsp honey
-2 Tbsp cilantro, chopped
-ground black pepper
For the garnish:
-1/4 cup fresh lime juice
-1 avocado
-1 small red onion, sliced thinly
-2 oranges, peeled and sectioned

Procedure:

In a large bowl, mix all of the ingredients with the exception of chicken. Make sure to coat the chicken well after adding it to the mixture and then cover the bowl and leave it in the fridge for 30 minutes.

Next, preheat the broiler or grill and take out the chicken from the marinade. Season with salt and pepper and make sure to discard the marinade.

Proceed to peeling and coring the avocado while the chicken is cooking. Make sure to chop it, as well. Mix it with the lime juice to avoid discoloration then add cilantro, orange, and onions.

Sprinkle salt all over the chicken and proceed to serving.

Enjoy!

Total Calories: 366

13.   Fishy Breezy Tacos

Ingredients:

-2 lbs cod fillets
-1 tomato, chopped
-juice of 2 limes
-1/4 tsp salt
-1/4 tsp black pepper
-1/4 tsp cayenne pepper
-1 tsp olive oil
-3 Tbsp cilantro, chopped
-1/2 onion, chopped
For the slaw:
-eight 6 inch corn tortillas
1/2 cup green onions, chopped
-2 cups red cabbage, shredded
-3/4 cup salsa
-3/4 cup non-fat sour cream
-2 cups red cabbage, shredded

Procedure:

First, preheat the oven to 350 °F.

Then, rinse the fish and put it on a baking dish rack so fat can be drained.

Combine onion, tomato, lime juice, cilantro, peppers, salt, and olive oil and spoon this mixture on top of the fillets. Cover with aluminum foil so fish could be moist then bake until flaky or for around 15 to 20 minutes.

Next, mix onion and cabbage together with salsa and sour cream and add it to the mixture that you have made earlier.

Make sure that fish has been divided equally among tortillas. Pour ¼ cup of the slaw on each fish tortilla and then fold to make tacos.

Serve and enjoy! Make sure to place leftovers in the fridge within 2 hours to keep them in good condition.

Total Calories: 180

14.   Poached Salmon served with Dill and Mustard Sauce

Ingredients:

-2 Tbsp shallots, chopped finely
-1 ¼ lb salmon fillet, skin on, cut into 4 portions
-1 tsp vegetable oil
-1/2 tsp salt
-1 ½ cup low-fat or fat-free milk
-1 ½ tsp cornstarch
-1 Tbsp fresh lemon juice
-2 tsp Dijon mustard
-1/4 cup reduced fat sour cream
-2 Tbsp fresh dill, chopped
-freshly ground black pepper, to taste
-fresh dill sprigs and lemon wedges, for garnish

Procedure:

Heat oil in a 10 inch skillet over medium heat before adding shallots. Sauté for around 30 to 60 seconds or until softened then add shallots, milk, salt, and pepper and let the mixture simmer, while stirring occasionally for around 10 to 12 minutes or until opaque.

Dip the salmon pieces in milk sauce then gently poach the salmon, covered. Spoon milk sauce occasionally over salmon and cook for another 10 to 12 minutes or until opaque.

Move salmon into another plate using a slotted spoon and then keep it warm by covering it with foil.

Then, mix cornstarch and lemon juice in a small bowl. Add this mixture to the milk sauce and cook for at least a minute, or until thick. Add mustard, chopped dill, and sour cream.

Serve garnished with dill sprigs and lemon wedges and with the dill and mustard sauce.

Total Calories: 338

15.   Grilled Chicken with Honey and Almonds

Ingredients:

-3 tsp honey
-1/4 cup Dijon Mustard
-1 tsp lemon juice
-4 skinless and boneless chicken breasts
-1/4 cup sliced almonds, toasted
-1 garlic clove, crushed

Procedure:

Preheat the broiler or griller and then blend lemon juice, honey, garlic, and mustard altogether in a small bowl.

Then, brush the chicken with the honey-mustard sauce that you have just made and then broil or grill for around 10 to 15 minutes away from heat source. Brush the chicken with some more sauce and discard the rest of the sauce.

Serve sprinkled with almonds. Enjoy!

Total Calories: 182

Chapter 4: DASH Diet Snack Recipes

16.   Blueberry-Lemon Oatmeal Muffins

Ingredients:

-1 cup all purpose flour
-1 ¾ cups oats, uncooked and divided
-1/2 cup granulated sugar
-2 Tbsp brown sugar, packed firmly
-1/4 tsp salt
-1 Tbsp baking powder
-1 tsp vanilla
-1 tsp lemon peel
-2 Tbsp vegetable oil
-2 lightly beaten egg whites
-1 cup fat-free milk
-1 cup blueberries, frozen or fresh

Procedure:

Heat the oven to 400 °F the place paper inside 12 muffin cups and then combine brown sugar with a cup of oats. Set this mixture aside.

Next, in a large bowl, mix 1 ½ cup oats with the rest of the ingredients. In another bowl, combine egg whites, vanilla, lemon peel, and milk and mix thoroughly.

Mix wet and dry ingredients together and stir until moist. Add berries and make sure to fill muffin cups until they are almost full.

Bake muffins until golden brown or for around 20 to 24 minutes and the let the muffins cool on a wire rack before serving. Make sure to serve warm.

Total Calories: 160

17.   Nacho Potatoes

Ingredients:

-2 tsp cooking spray
-1 lb small red potatoes, skins intact
-1/2 tsp chili powder
-8 oz 99% fat-free ground turkey
-1 cucumber, peeled and diced
-1 Tbsp cilantro, chopped
-1 medium tomato, diced
-1 cup lettuce, shredded
-1/2 cup cheddar cheese, shredded

Procedure:

Slice the potatoes into ¼ inch thick rings then coat them with oil.

Arrange the potato slices in a single layer on a baking sheet then bake for around 25 to 30 minutes at 400 °F.

Mix chili powder with ground turkey in a skillet. Cook for around 8 to 10 minutes or until browned and then take out the potatoes from the oven and place them in an oven-safe dish or on a casserole. Sprinkle cheese and ground turkey on top.

Then, bring the potatoes back to the oven and bake for around 2 minutes or until cheese melts. Take it out from the oven and mix with tomato, lettuce, cucumber, salsa and cilantro.

Serve and enjoy! Make sure to refrigerate leftovers within 2 to 3 hours.

Total Calories: 192

18.   Mini Zucchini Pizza

Ingredients:

-4 Tbsp pizza sauce
-4 large zucchini slices, cut into ¼ inch thick pieces
-2 Tbsp part-skim mozzarella cheese, shredded
-pepper, to taste
-cooking spray

Procedure:

Preheat the broiler to 500 °F then spray both zucchini sides with cooking spray and broil for 2 minutes per side.

Top each pizza slice with ½ tablespoon cheese and a tablespoon of pizza sauce then broil again until cheese melts or for another 1 to 2 minutes.

Serve immediately and enjoy!

Total Calories: 69

Ingredients:

-3 cups fat-free strawberry yogurt
-1 cup crunchy barley and wheat cereal
-1 cup light whipped topping
-1 cup fat-free condensed milk
-1 bag strawberries, ~~usweetened~~unsweetened

Procedure:

Sprinkle some cereal to the bottom of a lined baking pan and set aside.

Place strawberries, yogurt, and condensed milk in a blender and process until smooth.

Next, pour the strawberry and yogurt mixture on top of the cereal to smoothen the pan's edges. Freeze until firm or for around 8 hours.

Loosen foil to remove from the pan and thaw for at least 5 to 10 minutes before cutting into squares.

Serve topped with whipped cream, if desired. Enjoy!

Total Calories: 200

20.   Spiced Yogurt Pumpkin Pie Mix

Ingredients:

-1/2 cup pumpkin puree
-2 cups low fat plain yogurt
-1/4 tsp pumpkin pie spice
-1/4 cup walnuts, chopped
-1/4 tsp cinnamon
-honey/your choice of ~~sweeteer~~sweetener

Procedure:

Mix the pumpkin puree with the rest of the spices in a bowl then add yogurt ad mix thoroughly.

Put the mixture in serving dishes and top with walnuts and honey. You may use this not just for pumpkin pies, but also as dip for chips or nachos, if desired.

Enjoy!

Total Calories: 237

Chapter 5: DASH Diet Dessert Recipes

21.   Awesome Carrot Cookies

Ingredients:

-1/2 cup sugar
-1/2 cup packed light brown sugar
-2 eggs
-1/2 cup applesauce
-1/2 cup oil
-1 tsp ground cinnamon
-1 cup flour
-1 tsp vanilla
-1/2 tsp ground nutmeg
-1/4 tsp salt
-1 ½ cups carrots, grated finely
-2 cups rolled oats
-1/2 tsp ground ginger
-1 cup raisins

Procedure:

Preheat the oven to 350 °F.

Mix oil, eggs, applesauce, sugars and vanilla until well-blended.

Mix all of the dry ingredients together with the wet ingredients then add carrots and raisins.

Drop the mixture onto cookie sheets by spoonfuls. Bake until golden brown for around 10 to 12 minutes then store in an airtight container.

Enjoy!

Total Calories: 80

22. Nutty Blackberry Crumble

Ingredients:

-2 cups frozen or fresh blackberries
-1 Tbsp corn starch
-2 Tbsp sugar
-1/4 cup brown sugar
-1/4 cup all purpose flour
-1/2 cup rolled oats
-1 Tbsp diced unsalted butter
-1/8 tsp salt
-1/2 tsp cinnamon
-1/4 cup hazelnuts, chopped

Procedure:

Preheat the oven to 350 °F then coat a baking dish with cooking spray.

Combine cornstarch and sugar in a mixing bowl and mix until well-combined or until sugar has been incorporated in the mixture before adding lemon juice and berries. Stir until well-combined.

Next, pour the berries into a baking dish and scrape out any excess starch or sugar.

Combine flour, oats, brown sugar, salt and cinnamon in another bowl and mix well. Add butter and mix with the rest of the ingredients. Stir until crumbly before adding chopped hazelnuts.

Then, spread this mixture over the blackberries and bake for around 30 minutes in the oven.

Make sure to serve warm.

Total Calories: 240

23.   Strawberry and Pear Trifle

Ingredients:

-2 Tbsp lemon juice
-2 pears, pared and cored
-1/2 tsp almond extract
-2 cups strawberries, chopped coarsely
-1/2 9 inch angel food cake, cut into cubes
-2 Tbsp honey
-2 Tbsp orange juice
-3 cups lemon or vanilla flavored yogurt
-mint sprigs and pear slices

Procedure:

Toss pears and strawberries in almond extract and lemon juice and mix with honey and orange juice. Mix thoroughly.

Arrange 1/3 angel food cake with orange juice, a cup of yogurt, a cup of pear slices and a cup of strawberries. Repeat with the remaining ingredients.

Then, layer the rest of the cake with orange juice and a cup of yogurt. Refrigerate while covered with plastic wrap for around 1 to 4 hours then garnish with mint ad pear slices.

Serve and enjoy!

Total Calories: 161

24.   Fantastic Figs

Ingredients:

-2 Tbsp hot water
-1/4 cup orange juice
-1/3 cup sugar
-1/2 cup walnuts, chopped
-16 oz dried figs, stemmed and chopped
-1/2 tsp baking soda
-1 ½ cups all-purpose flour
-1 large egg
-1 cup packed brown sugar
-1/2 cup margarine, softened

Procedure:

Preheat the oven to 350 °F and make sure to spray a baking pan with oil.

Mix walnuts, figs, orange juice, hot water and sugar in a bowl before setting it aside. Beat brown sugar and margarine until creamy and then add the egg.

Then, combine baking soda with flour and mix with the egg mixture. Add oats so you could create some kind of soft dough. Make sure to reserve a cup of the said dough for the topping. Crumble this portion.

Press dough into the bottom of the pan and place the fig mixture on top. Then, add crumbled reserved dough on top but make sure that the fig mixture is visible.

Bake until golden brown or for around 30 minutes then let the mixture cool in a baking pan. After cooling, cut into bars and serve.

Make sure to refrigerate the leftovers within 2 hours.

Enjoy!

Total Calories: 125

25.   Berry Bowl Mash served with Frozen Yogurt

Ingredients:

-1 cup fresh blueberries
-1 cup strawberries, sliced
-1 cup fresh raspberries
-1 pint plain frozen yogurt
-3 Tbsp fresh orange juice
-1 tsp orange zest, grated
-1 Tbsp sugar

Procedure:

Mix sugar and berries in a bowl then remove zest from the orange with the use of a fine grater. Mix berries with the zest.

Then, slice the orange in half to get some juice out. Mix juice with the berries and toss until well-combined.

Place the mixture in the fridge for around 2 hours or overnight, if desired.

Place yogurts into some dessert bowls and add mashed berries on top.

Serve and enjoy!

Total Calories: 260

Conclusion

Thank you for reading this book!

I hope this book was able to open up your eyes about the beauty of the Dash Diet and have learned amazing recipes that you can make in order for you to live a great and healthy lifestyle.

The next step is to make sure that you didn't just read this book, but you took what you've learned to heart and that you'll really try making the recipes mentioned here.

Finally, if you have enjoyed this book, please don't forget to post a review on Amazon. It will be greatly appreciated!

Thank you and Good Luck!